Beyond Cancer Treatment

Beyond Cancer Treatment

*Clearing and Healing the
Underlying Causes*

DALE FIGTREE PhD

A Personal Memoir and Guide

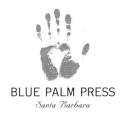

BLUE PALM PRESS
Santa Barbara

Published by Blue Palm Press
P O Box 61255, Santa Barbara, CA 93160, USA
studiokarts@earthlink.net

Design/production by Margaret Dodd, Studio K Communication Arts
Printed in the United States of America

The author neither makes nor attempts to make any diagnosis or cure or prevent
any disease. The author will not accept responsibility for any loss, injury or damage
caused or allegedly caused, directly or indirectly, by the information contained
in this book. The purpose of this book is to share her story and information that she
has acquired over the years. It is your choice to follow any or all of this information.
If you are unsure, please check with your health care professional.

*This book is dedicated to my parents, who generously
supported what they did not understand,
to Joya for her love and her fire,
and to Dr. Gian-Cursio for the gift of knowledge and wisdom
that continues to seed and flourish.*

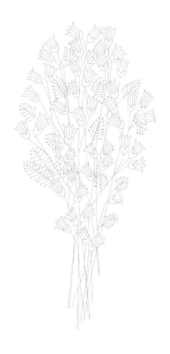

Eat Smarter: Smarter Choices for Healthier Kids
Health after Cancer
The Joy of Nutrition (DVD/video)

Section One: Healing Journey

Section Two: Healing Resources

Section One: Healing Journey

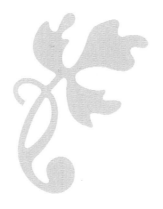

Foreword

*H*OW DO WE FIND OUR WAY HOME TO OUR SELVES, to a world of wholeness and meaning, when confronted by a life-threatening illness? In this refreshingly candid little book, Dale Figtree shares her odyssey of finding her way through the obstacles and challenges of diagnosis, treatment, cure and healing as she faces life-threatening cancer as a young woman of twenty-seven years.

The soul's story is not always easy to hear, it comes to us in bits and pieces, through dreams and synchronicities, through deep tears and agonizing sorrow as well as moments of joyful grace and miraculous healing. To listen to the deeper dimensions of life takes time that most of us in our hectic lives don't feel we have.

But those who have experienced or are facing life-threatening illness often have no choice. They are dragged into the depths of soul that we so studiously avoid in our fast-paced lives. They are the carriers of our contemporary healing myths, and we are blessed when they take the time to share their stories with us.

As a depth psychotherapist I know from years of experience that we can consciously participate in the life of the body, mind and soul if we choose to. But it takes time and hard work and may confront a patient with the need to challenge more conventional or acceptable healing routes. Deep attunement to the voice of one's own body may create a "difficult patient" for the medical profession. But as Dale points out, the difficult patient is often also the one who has the best chance of surviving a life-threatening illness. To fully participate in one's own healing process, she discovers, takes the attitude of the warrior.

But her story is more than just about surviving a life-threatening sentence; it is also about thriving and finding deeper meaning and a wider connection to life while living in the midst of confusion, doubt and crisis. She shows how the exploration of the underlying causes of her disease reveal healing opportunities. Like the mythical hero Odysseus she navigates through her own Scylla and Charybdis as she tackles the confusing array of healing approaches and advice and finds her way home to her own soul and body with its interconnectedness to ancestors and environment. In the process we are reminded that illness is a normal part of life and that the body itself has amazing healing capacities that we can either ignore or align ourselves with.

What I find especially admirable and significant is the total commitment with which Dale attunes herself to the interconnectedness of the physical, psychological and spiritual reality in which illness and healing takes place. In addition to traditional medical approaches and life-enhancing nutrition, she acknowledges the healing power of visualization, meditative practices and dream work. Determined to save her own life, she embraces the symbolic world of dreams, of mythic ritual, and creative expression, and she begins to notice that life responds with synchronicities, those acausal coincidences that create and reveal links between seemingly unconnected events or things. It was, she writes, "As if life was continuously presenting healing clues."

Intensely honest, the first part of her book is best read as memoir, a powerful healing story of what can happen when we move into relationship with the body from within its own reality. Dale discovers that the body may use crises and illness to clear toxins on physical, psychological and spiritual levels, and she reminds us that dreams may warn of an attitude to the embodied life that later shows up in disease. Never preachy or simply focused on cause and effect, she continually explores with respect and curiosity the synchronicities and "healing clues" that life brings when we dare to embrace illness from this deeply inclusive perspective.

Every person facing a life-threatening illness will have his or her own unique experiences, but Dale's story can serve as a well-informed guide, an Ariadne's thread to find one's way through the maze. For more concrete information she also adds a second part to the book that offers valuable nutritional and other healing resources that have been tested in the crucible of her experience.

> *Hendrika de Vries is a Jungian-oriented psychotherapist in private practice in Santa Barbara. She has been an adjunct faculty at Pacifica Graduate Institute, and a teacher, writer and presenter on the topic of Personal Mythology and Mythic themes in psychological and spiritual healing for over twenty years.*

Introduction

"When the time comes for the ego to set forth
on its journey towards wholeness,
strange and paradoxical things happen;
fate chooses strange emissaries.
But when we grow wiser we learn that the disasters of life
are often the genius of the unconscious,
forcing our egos into a new experience of the self."

Robert A. Johnson, from *We*

*I*N 1977, AT TWENTY-SEVEN YEARS OF AGE, I received the startling diagnosis of lymphatic cancer. Behind me, a cousin, an uncle, and a beloved grandmother—everyone I'd ever known or heard of with cancer—had died. There were no role models to cling to. And it wasn't just cancer, it was disease in general — if someone had diabetes, they eventually died of it; with arthritis it got worse; and heart disease—their days were numbered.

But in front of me, something new was in the air—slowly brewing—the potential for change. In retrospect I see it was not just for me, but was a collective shift beginning to happen. It was a shift towards deepening into exploring and developing our innate healing resources, and empowering ourselves to face life-threatening challenges in new ways, and in many instances, with new outcomes. We were beginning to birth a new age, where more of our vast capacity and self-healing potential was becoming available to us if we were willing to search for it.

And I was willing to search. I felt as though I had no choice—if I wanted to survive. This book is about that journey.

1

The Challenge

$\mathcal{I}$T CAME AS A SHOCK AT THE END OF EXTENSIVE treatment that the tumor in my left chest cavity was not entirely dissolved. I had been told that my particular type of malignancy, diffuse histolytic lymphoma, was responsive to radiation, and I had a chance for recovery if the cancer hadn't metastasized. This latest news, along with the fact that I had been exposed to the absolute lifetime limit of radiation in that area, left me terrified. It was then that I realized how very out of touch I had been with the reality of my situation, naively equating words like "responsive" and "recovery" with cure.

My oncologist, Dr. Jarowski, went on to explain that the lump in the X-ray, which had shrunk from a tumor the size of a grapefruit to the size of a grape, might possibly be just scar tissue. It could also, he explained, still have some malignancy left in it, in which case there was nothing else available except very extreme chemotherapy—and that would only slow down its growth. He felt that before initiating such drastic action, we should wait and see.

My symptoms had begun a few months earlier. I worked as a tapestry designer in a commercial studio filled with paints, solvents and other chemicals. After a long day of helping a colleague print designs on a large ink press reeking with fumes, I started to develop pains in my chest. Alarmed, that evening I headed for Emergency and got a chest X-ray. It revealed nothing unusual, and the pains gradually subsided by the next day. Within a month or two I developed a dry cough, an occasional pain near my left shoulder, and some odd feelings in my lungs. A doctor I consulted suggested I'd pulled a muscle and not to worry. Finally, six months after the initial X-ray, while visiting a friend in New York Hospital, I decided to get a second X-ray, as my symptoms seemed to be intensifying. This time the film revealed something completely blocking the left lung, and excess fluid filling my chest cavity. I was immediately hospitalized and put through two weeks of extensive testing, all of which proved inconclusive (before CT scans).

Finally, as a last diagnostic resort, I underwent

exploratory thoracic surgery, and a large cancerous tumor was discovered. It was in an advanced stage, pushing my heart to the other side of my chest and pressing closed my left lung. The tumor was considered inoperable due to its attachment, not only to my lung, but also to my heart and major arteries. A biopsy was taken and I was closed up.

During the procedure the nerve to my left vocal cord accidentally was severed, paralyzing that half of the cord and leaving me with literally half a voice—the higher half. Still, this seemed relatively minor compared to my other challenge.

2

The Vision

*T*HREE DAYS AFTER SURGERY, MY YOGA TEACHER and spiritual guide, Joya, paid a visit. She was a powerfully loving, wise and fierce individual. Sitting down on the bed, she looked me squarely in the eyes, and spewed forth the warning that I needed to "fight like hell" in order to survive. And part of the fight was to discover my influence in the creation of the cancer.

I was taken aback by her words, insinuating that I had something to do with creating this disease! Why would I ever want to create such a terrible situation? I felt I had a wonderful life! And when she spoke of fighting, I wasn't sure what she meant. After all, I was trying to keep a positive attitude and doing all that the doctors suggested. How else did one fight?

Before I could respond, she insisted that I lie quietly in the darkness and allow myself to go into a light meditation. Then as swiftly as she had appeared, she departed. After a few minutes, I released all thought, slipping into a semi-dreamlike state, and had the following vision.

Slowly forms appeared in a kind of micro-cellular landscape within my body. I could see cancer cells like slow-moving blobs with long sticky tentacles, lying chaotically in clusters at the bottom of a volcano-like structure. On a ridge above them, gathered in great masses, were strong white blood cells in the form of knights on horseback with great long lances, prepared for the onslaught. And suddenly, with a clash of cymbals, they came charging down, slicing, piercing, destroying each and every cancer cell until all was gone. Then sunlight began to filter in, illuminating the landscape, now filled with only pink healthy cells.

The image began to fade, and in that darkness another image slowly took form. It was of a child around five years of age, surrounded by her adoring family, at what seemed like a birthday party. I felt the little girl was me, although she didn't look exactly the way I looked as a child. The room was filled with wood and leather furniture from the 1940s, and a golden honey-colored light streamed in through the window. Then suddenly the image froze, cracked, and fell out, piece by piece, as though it were a broken mirror. And once again faded into darkness.

A subtle scent began to weave its way into my awareness—the smell of a forest—and then sound—of feet running through foliage—my feet—running up a hill through a group of people standing in a circle—finding my spot in the center and sitting down. There were three others seated and I was the fourth, completing the inner circle. As I sat I was able to look at myself as one looks in a mirror. I was a Mongolian youth—dark skin, black shiny hair, white teeth, and a strong body. There was a moment of stillness and then a great clash. Suddenly I found myself in the midst of a terrible war. Everyone was attacking each other using the most grotesque medieval flesh-ripping weapons, with blood spurting everywhere. Terrified, I felt at any moment I would be violently torn to pieces. My instinct was to leap and run for my life, but I would not budge. Somehow I knew I had prepared for this moment for a very long time, and was not to move. I had to sit and face my fear, face the possibility of a gruesome, painful death. And so I sat, my heart beating wildly, fear cutting through like a razor. After a few moments though, my heart began to slow down, my fear lessened, and my breathing eased. All that was outside of me gradually faded back into the darkness.

I then became aware of movement—of gliding quietly and swiftly through a dark tunnel. I sensed light at the far end, and found myself resisting and desperately not wanting to break through into that harshness. The closer I came to the light, the more I tried to resist, but to no avail—rather, the speed increased. Then suddenly, the light was upon me. Bracing myself, I tumbled through. My next sensation was of calmness, of floating free. I was in a brightly lit room—an operating room, looking down from the ceiling at a stillborn child that I knew had been me. And once again the image faded back into the darkness.

Then slowly a soft glow began to filter in, and I found myself sitting in a cave across from a sage-like male figure. I felt reverence being in his presence, and sensed we had an old, deep connection. I was unable to decipher his face as it kept changing too quickly, as though every face he had ever inhabited kept flashing by. We bowed graciously to each other, the tops of our heads touching, and in that moment I felt a river of ecstasy flowing into me from that spot. I became so intoxicated that I lost consciousness. When I awoke I found myself with my head comfortably resting upon his lap. Then, in a flash, he began to strike at my back with a hatchet. My first response was panic—to run—but then I realized the hatchet was not actually breaking my skin or even caus-

ing pain. It quickly dawned on me that he was attempting to kill something inside me, something I needed to get rid of. Fear turned into trust as I surrendered to simply being there. And then the image faded, and I lay awake in the darkness, reflecting on what I had just beheld.

All the images had meaning for me. The first one, of the micro-cellular landscape, was clearly about healing the cancer. I immediately recognized this as a powerful way to work with my illness—to imagine the healing process.

The second image of the child with adoring parents reminded me of a time when I was around five or six. For about a year I kept telling my mother that I had drowned. Needless to say, she was perplexed. The frozen frame and the pieces that fell out made me wonder if that was the child whose life was suddenly cut off—and if that child had been me in another life, if such a thing exists.

The third image of the Mongolian youth felt as though what I was about to face—"war"—involving my body, the cancer, and the treatment. I knew that my task was to be present and open to whatever transpired, even though another part of me desperately wanted to run. I sensed the boy also may have been me in another life, and that perhaps the initiation he had experienced was somehow connected to my present situation.

The fourth image of moving through the dark tunnel into the light is a strong collective out-of-body image that many people have reported experiencing. My resistance in the tunnel, and the dead infant at the other end, spoke to me of a death wish—of simply not wanting to be here. That was something I felt needed to be looked at carefully.

Even though I generally was excited about life and its vast potential, at the same time I had to acknowledge the existence of another side. Occasionally I would be seized by intense fear about the pain and horror of the darkest possibilities of existence, especially the thought of ever bringing a vulnerable child into such a threatening world. And in those moments, I simply did not know how I could go on. And then they would pass. Or would they just seep underground? I had to consider that having a life-threatening illness could be my way of escaping. Also, I wondered if this image and the image of the young girl whose life seemed to be cut off at five were attempts to incarnate in other lifetimes, where due to my resistance and fear of life, I didn't make it very far. And here I was, reaching a very precarious twenty-seven years of age. I couldn't help but think that perhaps this might be as far as I would get this time around.

The last image stirred me the most. It felt like being with my Spiritual Beloved. And then the merging—the fear and doubt—and the ease back into trust once again. Having this Being involved in my healing process helped me to have more faith in the enfoldment of what I was facing. He seemed to be watching over and working with me.

These images instilled in me a sense that having cancer was not just a matter of bad luck, but instead, an important part of my path, symbolic of deeper issues that needed to be seen, and ultimately healed.

3

Treatment

A FEW DAYS AFTER SURGERY, THE BIOPSY revealed that I had lymphoma—a cancer of the lymphatic system. I was started on radiation treatments with chemotherapy on the side. It never occurred to me that any other approach to healing existed. I trusted the doctors and did all they prescribed. The radiation treatments were painless in themselves, but an hour after each treatment I would develop a fever and fall into a deep sleep, awakening so drenched in sweat that my nightgown and sheets always needed to be changed. Within a few weeks my oncologist informed me that I was responding well, and the tumor had begun to shrink.

As for chemotherapy, I was initially told it could not

completely destroy this particular type of cancer, but that it hopefully would empower the radiation to work better. It was suggested that I do chemotherapy for three years, even though there was a 25 percent chance it might entirely knock out my hormonal system and throw me into premature menopause.

My attitude while in the hospital was actually very upbeat. During this time I really believed I would heal—after all, I was young, strong, and dedicated to a spiritual pursuit—things that I felt were sure to influence the outcome. Besides this, the truth of the matter was that I found the hospital fascinating. It was a large teaching hospital in the heart of New York City. I would wander around exploring different floors, and sun myself on the roof while viewing the Manhattan skyline. I was even asked to discuss the symptoms leading up to my diagnosis in a whole amphitheater of medical students.

On one of my walks through the corridors, wearing a red silk robe that I had purchased a few years before in San Francisco's Chinatown, a Chinese medical student stopped me. He asked if I knew the meaning of the large black Chinese character on the back of the robe, which of course I didn't. I was delighted when he revealed it meant "Long life!", a welcomed good omen.

After a few weeks in the hospital, I began to question certain things. I suspected that I was starting to be known as a "difficult patient." At one point, my oncologist came into my room wanting to do a procedure that required injecting dye into a lymph vessel in my foot. This would somehow "light up" my entire lymph system in order to check for any other enlarged lymph nodes or tumors. I remembered years back when my grandmother went through this same procedure and how afterwards she cried for days from the pain, so I refused to have it done and just took my chances. Then I was sent to a throat specialist to treat my paralyzed vocal cord. He wanted to inject latex into it in order to move it closer to the other vocal cord, giving me a more normal voice. Latex, in my cells, forever! "No thank you," I responded.

Then, after six weeks I was finally discharged from the hospital, though I continued to return each week for radiation and chemo. After the third month of treatment, my oncologist called me into his office to discuss my latest X-ray. He informed me of a newly discovered smaller mass, a few inches below the original tumor. His whole staff was in agreement that it was a second tumor, that the cancer had metastasized, and that radiation should begin on that new area the very next day. I went home panic-stricken! Up until this point, I emotionally resided in a simple, almost naive kind of optimism—trusting God, trusting my spirit guides, trusting the doctors, and trusting that my path was to heal. But now all of that was slashed in an instant, and the harsh reality of my situation hit home—that I might soon be facing a difficult death.

Once home, I immediately called Joya and blurted out the terrible news. She suggested that I sit down, right then, and meditate, and she would see me in a few days when she came back into town. As I attempted to sit with an agitated mind, I decided to use my imagination and recreate the first scenario of the vision from a few months before (something I had let slip by until this moment). Once again I pictured the cancer cells at the bottom of a volcano, and my immune cells lining up in droves of thousands and thousands, above. And with a clash of cymbals they charged down into the volcano, row after row. Then the destruction—as each wounded cancer cell evaporated—until the ground was filled with only healthy pink cells. As I slowly opened my eyes I found myself in a state of serenity. Something had happened—a gifting. My fear had mysteriously vanished! Afterwards, I was able to enjoy my dinner and even have a good night's sleep!

At the hospital the next morning, another X-ray was taken to calculate the exact measurements for the new area of radiation. A few minutes later, my oncologist entered the room looking baffled. He announced that the second lump was gone—vanished—a spontaneous whatever—even though the original tumor was still there. The doctors didn't quite believe it themselves and took another series of X-rays from different positions—but nothing was ever found, and radiation to this new area was never begun.

Astonishment! A miracle had truly happened with the visualization. And in a split second I was out of that immediate crisis. It was strange though, and very disorienting in that it had been so unexpected and so inexplicable. I felt definitely relieved and grateful, yet somehow I remained slightly detached emotionally. Considering what had just taken place, I thought that an odd reaction. Looking more closely, I realized there was an element of unrealness in all that was going on. I had never seen or directly felt the actual tumor. I did not feel the radiation treatments while they were being administered, though I was informed regularly that they were shrinking the tumor. Then I was told of a new tumor, and now I was told it was gone. It was strange, relying on secondhand information for potentially disquieting updates.

I also recognized that the only time I became truly emotionally involved was when I believed the threat of death was present. When that was no longer pressing, I seemed to slip back into a detached state again. Seeing this alarmed me, for I sensed it was important for my recovery to stay more involved, especially since the original tumor was still there. So I began to do visualization with the rest of my treatments, helping them along with mental images of the destruction of the cancer cells. This was the first time I had participated in the healing process other than just placing my body on the table and letting the machines do the work.

After a few more months of treatments, the radiation started to affect what was left of my voice, causing me to stutter at times and experience difficulty pronouncing certain words. Scar tissue was forming in my lungs where the radiation had burned away cells. My left lung started to contract and tighten due to the scarring, so that its capacity to hold air was diminishing.

In the meantime, the chemotherapy was causing my blood to become anemic, and my immune system dangerously depleted. My hair started to slowly thin and grow in a much fainter shade of color. I had begun to lose the natural reflexes in my feet and knees, and experienced a continual tingling in my fingertips and toes, which my oncologist explained as the destruction of nerve endings. I developed rashes on my arms and abdomen, and sores in my mouth. I noticed also, along with some of my friends, that I was becoming increasingly moody. And these were only the side effects that were most obvious! I was beginning to feel weak and sickly, yet I easily accepted that as being part of the price I had to pay to get well again.

Then one day, after four months of treatment, I

stumbled upon a book a housemate of mine, a pre-med student, had left lying on a table. The book was basically about laetrile, but also described in great detail the inadequacies and hidden dangers of conventional medical treatments for cancer: radiation, surgery and chemotherapy. The more I read, the more disturbed I became at the statistics and the degree of damage associated with these treatments, the dark side that doctors usually don't talk about and that I didn't ask about! I had no idea these treatments were, in so many instances, so devastating to the body. One of the most frightening parts of the book was reading about reactions from the three specific drugs that I was taking, as the book described story after story of things gone terribly wrong. Even worse were the damage and failure rates of radiation treatments: how the majority of the tumor was easily destroyed, but how the core, the last 5 percent, contained the most potent part of the malignancy, and was in many cases impossible to eradicate.

The radiation was practically over, so there was not much to be done about that, but I wanted to talk to my oncologist as soon as possible about getting off chemotherapy, and discuss other less damaging approaches to healing. I tried telephoning him but his line was busy. Literally five minutes after I put the phone down, it rang, and lo and behold, my oncologist was on the other end of the line! He had just come from a meeting with his staff, and they unanimously decided to take me off all chemotherapy, right away, explaining only that it was not having the desired effect on the tumor. I was relieved at the speed with which my desire to get off the drugs had been implemented, and once again was amazed at the synchronicity of events as they unfolded.

After six months, I had reached the limit of radiation I could have in that area and the treatments were stopped. I needed to wait a month to let the results settle and then took my final X-rays. I was looking forward to the results, marking the end of my treatment.

When my oncologist called me into his room, his face appeared dark and serious. I could not believe my ears when he told me the tumor had been reduced by about 90 percent but was still not entirely gone. I found this incredulous, sounding just like the book described! Surely he could operate and take out what was left, but he explained that due to radiation damage, the tissues would fall apart. I enquired about new trials, new experimental drugs, anything—but he just looked sullen, and said as far as he knew, there was no other medical approach left to dissolve the tumor completely.

I was stunned and felt abandoned—suddenly on my own in all of this. And it was a terrifying yet magnificent moment, for it was then that I was shaken awake to the desperate need to save my own life.

This feeling of urgency, not a moment to lose, created a laser-like focus. That intensity found a voice through inwardly asking, praying, petitioning for guidance and help. And almost immediately, a whirlwind of information, insights, books, synchronicities and helpful people began to pour into my life. It was amazing, as if life was continuously presenting healing clues! Perhaps it had always been, but I wasn't tuned in or sensitive enough to notice. I knew I needed to pay close attention to all that was being offered, and then explore those things with discrimination, gathering carefully what would be the most valuable modalities to incorporate into my healing process. It felt like creating an alchemical container, which is filled with certain carefully chosen ingredients, then sealed and cooked and cooked—like a pressure cooker. When it's time to open the container back up, hopefully a transformation of healing will have taken place. That was what I was going for.

4

New Healing Resources

*T*HE PATH OF MY HEALING WORK SOON BEGAN TO clarify. The first thing that seemed most important to deal with was my "will to live." I felt if I was going to fight for my life, I needed to "want to live" for a powerful reason, other than just fear of death. But to my surprise, almost bewilderment, when I looked deeply into what that was, I found nothing really held that much importance. I was somewhat ambivalent towards the things that most people yearn for—marriage, children, and professional success. I had come of age during the late 60s—a time when a whole generation shifted from society's accepted patterns to exploring what was more relevant and true for them. I jumped right in, experiencing many different facets of life as I traveled abroad for several years, and finally ended up in New York City, embracing a spiritual path. Yet in the end, somehow all of this, still, was not enough to passionately want to live for.

During the next few days I experienced the discomfort of nothing to really hold on to, then slowly I began to make contact with a deeper aspect of myself, one that holds a rich appreciation for simply being a part of this complex, mysterious, sacred world. I was able to feel the gifting of having a life, a body, an opportunity to experience and explore, inwardly and outwardly—the amazement of it all. I found myself making a deal, so to speak, with Spirit—to live out my potential to the greatest degree I am capable of, and to open as wide as possible to the fullness of it all. With intent and probably a lot of grace, I somehow was able to cut through a layer of numbness and discover a strong connection to life.

Once I was able to feel that rich connection, I knew I needed to deal with a part of me that held a possible death wish. It was something I was slowly beginning to see more clearly. It was also what Joya seemed to be pointing out, in regard to a hidden subtle sense of overwhelm and fear of the pain of life. Upon recognizing it, I knew that the part of me wanting to live was stronger and larger than the part that wanted to escape. I somehow suspected that the desire to escape seemed to have more power and danger if it lurked undetected, slipping through the shadows. So I paid closer attention when it came up, even as a slight passing thought or feeling. Many times, by examining layer after layer of what I wanted to run away from, it would transform into a valuable insight.

Then there was the fear of dying I needed to work with. (It was odd being sandwiched between fear of living and fear of dying.) I knew intense fear about the cancer and death could freeze me and become a negative force. Yet I also knew a certain amount of fear was natural and even appropriate for this situation, instilled in all living creatures as a survival instinct. So instead of just trying to defuse my fear, I learned to accept it and even put it to use. I've come to appreciate that fear can be a wonderful mechanism to sharpen one's awareness and cause actions to have greater force behind them. Times when I was gripped with fear, I would parlay that intensity into my daily visualization work and meditation practice, which served to enhance and empower it—like rocket fuel.

The next step was about recognizing how I had not fully acknowledged the cancer, and had given responsibility of my healing completely over to the doctors. This insight motivated me to look at everything I did, from staying up late at night to drinking a glass of wine. I began to question everything—EVERYTHING—

whether it contributed to my recovery or not! If not, then it was put on the shelf, hopefully until I was out of this crisis. I became careful how I lived my life. This acknowledgement of the cancer felt like a big break-through.

The obvious next step was to focus on visualiza-tion—especially considering the profound experience of the second tumor disappearing. I devoted time each morning and evening, and sometimes in the afternoon, to this practice. The intensity of my situation helped keep this work always sharp and fresh, instead of becoming habitual and boring. As each day passed, my faith grew stronger in the power of one's deeper will, and the healing power of the Divine.

I began to become more and more creative during my visualization sessions. At one point I had the sense to place a beautiful organic apple I had just purchased on my meditation table, and to breathe any dis-ease left in my body into the apple. Then I felt guided to bury the apple. Grabbing a big spoon, I went out into the garden of my rented house, and there in front of a statue that I thought was Saint Francis, I dug deep and buried the apple. I then asked the Earth to accept the apple as a substitution sacrifice instead of my body, which I acknowledged would ultimately go back to the earth anyway—though hopefully later than sooner! After-wards, as I was driving with a friend, we passed a hospital displaying the same statue on top of the roof as I had in my garden. I blurted out, "There's Saint Francis." My friend, who was much more astute in such matters, corrected me. "That's not Saint Francis, that's Saint Anthony, the Patron Saint of Healing!" Tingles went down my spine!

During this time, perfect books came my way. Two of them, *Journey to Ixlan* and *Tales of Power* by Carlos Castaneda, seemed to speak to me about things I needed to recognize and act upon in my process of becoming well. His teacher Don Juan spoke about the "Path of the Warrior"—living life with razor-sharp awareness, especially the awareness of the possibility of death always close by, as it gives one's acts greater power, as if each act might be the last. He also spoke about how to recognize clues that life constantly presents to us, guiding us for answers to our questions and prayers, sometimes simply re-affirming that we are moving in the right direction, or perhaps warning us that we are headed for trouble. He put into words exactly what I had started to experience once I asked for help. Each time I read from these books, my energy somehow shifted and I would find myself in an expanded state of consciousness for the next hour or two.

I also read the *Ramayana*, a major ancient Hindu myth. It is the story of the Great Spirit who incarnates on earth in the form of a prince called Rama, along with his princess, Sita, to clean up widespread corruption. Their greatest devotee, Shiva, incarnates also, in order to be of service, and appears in the form of a humble glorious monkey called Hanuman, who ultimately saves the day. The story is rich with symbolism and deep relevant truths about life. I was so delighted by it that I decided to create a life-size clay bust of Hanuman as a gift for Joya. My work on this statue filled me with great satisfaction and actually felt as nourishing as all my other healing practices.

5

Nutritional Support

*F*INALLY, IT WAS TIME TO DEAL WITH THE PHYSICAL —to find out what my body needed to get strong and healthy, to correct the malfunction that had allowed the cancer to grow in the first place, and to clean out toxicity and heal any damage done by the chemotherapy and radiation.

A friend suggested I see a doctor she knew and highly respected, Cristopher Gian-Cursio, a doctor of Natural Hygiene and Naturopathy. He had directed many people on food programs for several decades, and had a reputation for remarkable cures of various degenerative diseases, including cancer.

During our first telephone conversation, after telling him about my health situation, he quickly ended the conversation, telling me to call his secretary for an appointment. I called the next day, and the next, and the next, leaving messages, but never got a call back. It took a month of perseverance—of calling every single day—until I wore him down and he finally agreed to set up an appointment. First though, he insisted I see an associate of his, an old-time medical doctor who was about ninety years old. The doctor made a few taps here and there, and took an X-ray with an antique machine. In the end he gave me a stamp of approval and invited me to come back in ten years to share a bottle of champagne with him—what a sense of humor!

When finally Dr. Cursio and I did meet, I saw in his face the gravity of my situation—something the staff at the hospital had mostly managed to keep hidden. He gave me no encouragement or positive feedback about the possible results of doing his program. He didn't even suggest I come back. I left feeling terrible, but determined. He wasn't going to get rid of me that easily!

It wasn't until much later that I discovered the reason behind his hesitation to treat me. Apparently several years earlier Dr. Cursio had been arrested four different times for treating people who had cancer. The medical climate at that time was stifling, as it was actually illegal to treat cancer any other way than by chemo, surgery or radiation! Unbeknownst to me, he was taking a risk having me as a client.

Dr. Cursio prescribed a food program containing a huge amount of fresh, unadulterated foods. He explained that an abundant amount of high nutrients would give my body the fuel and raw materials to do deep cleansing, rebuilding and rebalancing. Although I didn't completely understand his system at that time, I followed his instructions as closely as I could. I knew there was no guarantee that this diet or anything else I was doing would save my life, but if I didn't try "110 percent," what was the point!

Along with food choices, rest was also a major priority. Energy needed to be conserved to be more available for the deeper healing work. Dr. Cursio said that there would be a time, further down the line, to jump back into a strong exercise program, but for the present, freeing up the energy to be used as the body best wants to use it was crucial.

Within a week I developed a severe cold, coughing up large amounts of mucus with what looked like tiny black threads in it. Dr. Cursio advised me to stay in bed, drink fresh vegetable juices, and let the symptoms run their natural course. I did not believe it would be possible for me to get through a cold without a decongestant, but I somehow managed. I suspect that not having any dairy or wheat products in my diet contributed to less clogging.

Shortly after that I developed diarrhea for a few

days, which cleared up by itself. Even though I was eat-ing enormous quantities of food, my weight began to drop and I began to weaken.

After a month I requested a follow-up appointment. When Dr. Cursio asked how I was feeling, I lied, reporting instead that I felt great. Because of his initial hesitancy in seeing me, I feared he might drop me if he heard I was not doing well on the program. Oddly, he didn't seem pleased with my response.

The next month passed with more weight loss and even greater weakness. Just walking up stairs left me breathless. I was beginning to get scared, so that when I saw Dr. Cursio for the third time, I couldn't hold back—blurting out how bad I felt, despite the feared consequences. But much to my surprise, he lit up and he literally shouted, "Wonderful!" He explained that finally my body appeared to be responding and clean-ing itself out. He said that the discomfort was due to toxic wastes being emptied. The weakness was due to energy being pulled from my muscles to be used instead for deep reparative work. He assured me, when this work was completed, my energy would return. It made sense, and I felt relieved and hopeful.

After this, my relationship with Dr. Cursio changed. He seemed genuinely happy to see me on my monthly visits, and at times even took me under his wing, show-ing me his vast collection of out-of-print books from the great "Natural Hygiene" doctors of the past. He would always take time to carefully answer my many questions about the workings of particular foods or symptoms. Little did I know that those times were the precious beginning of my education in the healing arts.

After another month my weight was down from 120 to 105 pounds. Losing 15 pounds is frightening for someone who just had cancer. Interestingly though, it was the exact amount I had originally lost during my six-week stay in the hospital. Then when I returned home, I found that I had an obsessive need to stuff myself with food—any food until my stomach literally cried out in pain. I regained the 15 pounds within a few weeks. Now, on my new food program, those 15 pounds seemed the first thing to be flushed out. Much to my surprise, Dr. Cursio did not seem concerned— on the contrary, he felt it was progress—part of clearing out unhealthful tissue and toxins. He simply encouraged me to be patient, and seemed confident that the weight would return as healthier, stronger tissue. Sure enough, five months into the program, on the exact amount of food, not only did I regain every single pound, but I even started to put on a little extra.

It took me years before I understood this had nothing to do with calories, as my diet was actually rich in calories. It was the high levels of nutrients that fired up my metabolism, and in turn, my body had the power to do intensive breaking down and cleaning out of unhealthful tissue and accumulated toxic material or waste, which was the true reason for the weight loss. Dr. Cursio also explained that my intestines were literally being scraped clean of old mucousy, decayed material by high fiber foods, causing absorption levels to rise. At a certain point my system was cleared, so that the rebuilding process could dominate. This, along with better absorption of nutrients, caused my weight to increase to its most healthful place.

During this time I also experienced a variety of different symptoms—headaches, aches and pains, nausea, sore throats, and so on. I was beginning to recognize that many of these common symptoms are simply an exaggeration of the body's normal actions, intensified to have greater force to work on or push out something the body wants to be rid of. The way I looked at colds and flu and other so-called illnesses changed. I recognized that they also intensify remedial actions of the body, cleansing, repairing, healing, and then restoring balance.

Besides all of this, I also was slowly getting my full voice back. My closest friend Angani was a wonderful singer/songwriter, and we spent many hours singing our hearts out together. I was hoping that if anything would help realign my vocal cords, singing would— and it seemed to be working!

These months were actually a very special and critical time. Joya had gone to India for several months, and other close friends had moved away. Suddenly I found myself more alone and without distraction—something that took a while to get used to. Everything I did was becoming a part of my healing process.

My days consisted of preparing and eating food, which took a long time, especially in the beginning while becoming accustomed to making everything from scratch. The worst part was cleaning the juicer three times a day. This in particular annoyed me, but was quickly resolved by paying my housemate's thirteen-year-old daughter to wash the juicer. All was well until a month later when she left for a vacation, returning the cleaning chore back to me. As I begrudgingly scrubbed away, I suddenly had a rich insight—that everything I did connected to food was actually part of my healing process. The more I did, the more intensified the process became—even cleaning the juicer. With that awareness, all resistance fell away and I embraced cleaning the juicer and all else encompassed in my healing routine as empowering my chances for getting well.

Between this and all the other healing modalities I had gathered into my life, the container was full and concentrated. Intermittent fears about the future would occasionally freeze me and drag down my spirit, but as

soon as I became aware of it, I'd work with those feelings, and sooner usually than later, I'd be back in the
present moment where I was alive and powerfully
connected to a creative healing process.

6

Dreams

ANOTHER RICH PART OF MY HEALING CONTAINER was dreams. As I was about to record a dream that seemed relevant to my situation, I stumbled across another dream I had written down, from over two years before.

I am with a Hindu Holy man named Sai Baba. He wants to reach inside my chest and pull out something the size of a marble. At first I am agreeable, but then I begin to have resistance, questioning him about the anesthetic and the antiseptic. In the end, I refuse his help.

I couldn't believe what I was reading—that two years before the tumor was discovered in the exact same place, Sai Baba, or whomever he represented in my dream, seemed to know something was there—and I wouldn't let it be removed! At that time I was suffering from walking pneumonia, which seemed to go on and on, which I developed shortly after cleaning up flea powder (without wearing a mask) that I had spread throughout my whole apartment.

Sai Baba was known to me only from a photograph my meditation teacher kept on her table. He was a great spiritual teacher in India and had a reputation for healing his devotees through dreams. I was faced with the cruel realization that I might not have had to go through all of this. This ate away at me for days until I came to terms with it—accepting that my path was to go through this experience with its lessons, and hopefully grow and be changed by it—for the better.

Many of my dreams have been coherent and meaningful throughout my life, and effortlessly remembered, as far back as age five. During this challenging time, my dreams began to reflect what I sensed was reaffirming the modalities I chose to work with, and pointing in the direction of healing.

One of the first dreams I had during this concentrated healing time had to do with Hanuman, the great monkey devotee from one of the books I was reading, the *Ramayana*. My teacher Joya had spoken about him, and strangely, when I was in the hospital, there was a subtle design in the ceiling texture that looked just like Hanuman's face—as though this mythological figure was watching over me.

I am opening up a letter that has come to me from India. Inside are two pictures of Hanuman. I am fascinated by the beautiful colors of each picture. One is bright and colorful, where he is a fierce and powerful warrior. The other picture has muted, subtle tones, showing Hanuman as a loving devotee, pulling his heart open—revealing the presence of the Divine living inside.

As the dream ends I am awakened by a knock on my door. It is my housemate, who hands me a letter that has just arrived from a friend traveling in India. To my amazement it contained the two pictures of Hanuman that I had just dreamt about. What synchronicity! I accepted these pictures as a special gift that could very well be connected to my healing process. To this day I keep them on my meditation table. It was after this dream that I decided to make a life-size bust of Hanuman as a gift to Joya. This work also became a part of my healing container.

The next dream followed a few weeks later.

I am with a few friends, standing on a cliff overlooking a long stretch of beach that winds around like a crescent for miles and miles. Far in the distance are clouds of sand, stirred up by the galloping horses of the enemy that appears to be on its way to attack us. I go into our house on the cliff where a flurry of activity is taking place—cleaning guns, making ammunition, and building barricades. We are scared, but we are brave and prepared to fight if we have to, rather than retreat. At one point, a friend approaches and asks for a tray of ammunition. I hand him a platter filled with clay bullets, the same sort of cylindrical shapes I make of my clay before applying it to the Hanuman statue I am working on. As it turns out, the enemy never comes.

The "enemy" not showing up in the dream felt synonymous with the cancer not coming back. The similarity with the clay cylinders I used as I made the Hanuman statue and the ammunition to stop the enemy seemed to suggest that my creative work might be contributing to my healing. I've come to appreciate through the years the role creative expression plays in healing with many people I've met, artists and non-artists alike. Besides having a nourishing aspect, it also seems to give a voice to hidden forces within that may powerfully affect the healing process.

Another dream appeared shortly after.

I am adrift in a small rowboat with no oars on a great sea with nothing in sight. Suddenly, a big ocean liner appears on the horizon and rescues me. I am taken directly to the dining room, starved. With my mouth watering, I closely eye several large cakes, thick with icing, inside a glass case. A waiter appears and asks to take my order. I straighten up and say, "I would like a big salad, please."

Drifting in a small boat on a great ocean is a fairly common image dying people have as they are slipping away towards death. Being rescued by a big ocean liner may indicate that life-saving help comes in the form of large energy—possibly team support rather than a singular person or way.

Choosing a salad over all the tempting deserts feels like moving past the superficial and immediate gratification to something certainly more substantial and real—giving up a kind of childhood innocence. Also, connecting being rescued with eating a salad reinforces nutrition as a powerful healing tool.

After a few weeks another dream appeared.

I am at a spiritual retreat talking to Joya's assistant, a woman named Kali Maha, about activating the defense mechanisms in my body. Next I go to the hospital to get a transfusion. The nurse inserts a needle into the vein of my right hand, and then departs. I decide to leave before the transfusion is complete, thinking I'll return later to get it done. Then I am with Joya. I say to her, "There is only a pea-size piece of cancer left in my body, only a damn pea!" She responds, "Open your shirt and let me pluck it out." I protest, saying, "No, I'll do it." She says, "Don't be a fool. Let me." I stubbornly again refuse, but then it occurs to me that if I truly could pluck out the cancer, it wouldn't still be there. In the end I surrender and accept Joya's healing offer. I open my shirt and she reaches into my chest cavity and pulls out the pea, and says, "There!"

Looking at the dream, I wondered if this could be a second chance to accept healing help. This time I let Joya, who perhaps represents Feminine Energy or even my inner healer, remove the tumor, something I would not let Sai Baba (perhaps representing the Masculine) do in the dream from two years earlier. I awoke realizing that I might actually be healed—that during the dream, what was left of the cancer may truly have been removed from my body.

In the beginning of the dream, leaving the hospital before the transfusion is complete suggests something other than what the doctors have to offer is required for my full healing. That I had part of the transfusion may indicate that the medical route contributed to a part of my healing process. Also, deciding myself to leave is taking decisions into my own hands, which goes along with being considered a "difficult patient." Several years later I came across the book *Love, Medicine and*

Miracles, in which Bernie Siegel suggests that "difficult patients" tend to be survivors more so than compliant ones. Challenging authority is also about challenging the father/daughter or teacher/student relationship— instead of wanting approval, the concern is stronger to follow one's truth no matter what.

7

Next Phase

Six months after I was discharged I went back to see my oncologist for a follow-up X-ray and blood work. When I entered his office to hear the results, he was beaming. According to my blood test, I was his healthiest patient. And my X-rays, although they were becoming increasingly difficult to read due to scar tissue from the radiation, seemed to suggest that the grape-sized lump in my chest had not changed. My doctor thought this was a very good sign, since the cancer had been highly malignant and fast-growing. He confessed that when he discharged me previously, he did not feel very optimistic about my prognosis, but now he seemed delighted and genuinely positive about my future. He wanted to know "what the heck" I was doing. I explained to him about the food regime and visualization, but I could see it really wasn't registering. As we parted he patted me on the back, and simply encouraged me to continue whatever I was doing — something appeared to be working!

Walking out of the office, I felt elated — the greatest challenge in my life seemed to be successfully resolving. Little did I know this was just the tip of the iceberg.

A month later I moved from New York City to Joya's ranch community in Roseland, a rural part of Florida. Within a short time, everyone there (about 150 people), including Joya, was working with Dr. Cursio. He flew down once a month and spent two days seeing one person after another, giving each their own specific food plan for the month. These times proved a rich source for gaining more understanding about the variations of his food programs and the healing processes that seemed to be triggered by them.

It soon became obvious that each person's progress was unique though, for the most part, the majority of people at the ranch were considered cleaned out or detoxified after nine months. Most felt healthier and more energized than they had previously, without having to go through too much discomfort. Yet a few other people, who didn't appear unhealthy, were having much more extreme physical reactions as their bodies cleaned out, especially compared to what I had gone through. The doctor had always spoken of a powerful major healing crisis that some people must go through before truly re-establishing strong health, and it seemed as though that hadn't happened to me yet, even though I intermittently experienced minor "cleansing" symptoms.

When Dr. Cursio witnessed a dinner at the ranch, with everyone juicing and blending—and big platters of steamed vegetables and so on, tears came to his eyes. His knowledge and great gifting had manifested on a scale he never imagined. And for me, that the food I originally spent hours each day preparing was now there for the taking, was a gift beyond measure.

8

Transformation

*A*FTER THREE RELATIVELY QUIET YEARS healthwise, one day without any cold or upper respiratory symptoms, I started coughing up "golf-ball-size" globs of mucus, to such a degree that I found myself choking at times. A few weeks later I had difficulty focusing my eyes, seeing black spots wherever I looked. Shortly after, I developed a fever, 104 degrees F. for a few days, then down to a steady 102 degrees F. I was experiencing extreme aches and stiffness in my joints and my pulse rate sped up to a constant 140 beats per minute. On top of all of this, I also had drenching sweats that smelled similar to the odor from sweats during radiation treatments.

Soon after, I developed a pain so intense in the area

where I previously had cancer that I could not lie still for more than a few minutes day or night without writhing in agony. Although I was committed otherwise, I was constantly tempted to take pain medication. Amritha, a chiropractor visiting the ranch, did a few adjustments to my back, which helped ease some of the pain. Also, I noticed if I pressed strongly into the area of discomfort, it became numb after a while. So I asked a friend to bring me a tennis ball and cut it in half. I placed one half directly under the most painful spot and pressed my weight into it, and was able to stay pain-free for long stretches of time—"homemade acupressure!" After a few weeks the pain decreased to the point where I could even forget about it at times without having to do anything.

A few days into the fever I also developed diarrhea, which lasted about six weeks. My weight began to drop and after one month I lost 10 pounds, even though I was still managing to eat three large meals a day. The symptoms, though slightly reduced, were still fairly intense. My fever wavered at between 102 and 101 degrees F. I had never met anyone who had a fever for a month, nor had a doctor who lived on the ranch, Dr. Harry, who was keeping a watchful eye over me. He authorized testing, which revealed nothing specific. X-rays showed the lump was still present, but appeared not to have changed, and blood tests and sputum cultures ruled out pneumonia and other infections.

Dr. Cursio felt this was my big purge—an opportunity to empty whatever was underlying the cancer in the first place, along with the debris left over from my treatment. He advised complete bed rest, lots of high-nutrient food, and patience.

After two months there was still no significant change, except that I dropped another 10 pounds. At the end of the third month the symptoms were still going strong, and my weight had slipped to barely 90 pounds. By this time I caught wind of the fact that most of the people on the ranch thought I was dying of cancer. A friend who came to visit from New York burst into tears when she walked into my room. Joya, though, had a kind of "knowing" twinkle in her eye when she saw me, encouraging me to just hang in there.

Of course I was frightened that the cancer might have returned, but was also aware Dr. Cursio could be correct—that this might be my major healing crisis, and could mean finally being cleaned out, healed, and truly healthy. From the start of the symptoms, I considered both sides. I knew that if I saw a cancer specialist I would instantly be put in the hospital and given toxic tests and drugs that would start the body poisoning all over again—and to what end? I felt I'd worked too hard for that. The results from the testing certainly helped give me extra courage, and so I held on tight to the belief that I was going to recover. I decided to just let it unfold without interfering.

After resolving that, I was able to rest in a kind of revelry, sleeping a lot and reading two books a friend had brought me. Both were by a woman named Taylor Caldwell on the lives of Jesus and St. Paul. Not having been raised Christian, I knew little of the detail of these stories, but as I read, tears flowed and my heart was continually touched. For those months I lay bathed in a soft sweet essence that I imagined might be connected to Jesus and his life and teachings.

During the third month of symptoms, a friend mentioned an incident that had happened the night before at a ranch gathering. A woman stood up and spoke about her concern that I was not doing enough. Joya lashed out at her, saying she had no right to judge me, and no idea what I was going through and the work that was being done. Somehow hearing this was a reminder that perhaps I could do more. I had let go of my visualization practice, feeling too uncomfortable to sit or do any inner work. But suddenly I remembered its potency, and I restarted visualizing healing light pouring through my body. One night as I sat to meditate and do a healing visualization, I kept nodding off to sleep. After about 40 minutes of struggling, as I was repeatedly pulling myself back to present awareness, a jolt of energy shot through my body, and I found myself completely awake and highly energized. I did my visualization and then attempted to go to sleep, but the energy was so strong and so alive in my body that I simply did not sleep at all that night. Once again I felt the possibility that this energy could be a gift of healing, somehow connected to my willingness to persevere.

By the fourth month there was still no let-up of symptoms. I had become so weak that even bathing myself became difficult. I was so thin and boney that my knees hurt from pressing into each other when I slept on my side. I remember being able to slide a normal size bracelet past my elbow all the way up my arm. At this point, Dr. Harry was panicking, and was pushing for hospitalization. Amritha, my chiropractic friend, fought this, feeling that in my weakened condition, I could pick up any germ or bacteria. Dr. Harry suggested instead that I take a round of strong antibiotics, in the hope that it would put a stop to the symptoms. I felt between a rock and a hard place. I had to admit the state of my body was becoming frightening, so I hesitatingly agreed, and took antibiotics for ten days. Nothing happened. Nothing changed. Finally, Dr. Harry suggested I summon my parents. Though he hadn't put words to it, I got that he thought any day I could be gone. That really shocked me, yet once again connected me to the severity of my situation. Even if I was just detoxifying, it suddenly hit me that I could still slip away.

That realization shook me, and once again I felt a powerful urgency to evoke change. First I decided to double the amount of food I was eating, although I was already eating normal-size portions. Then I went inside, and with all the ferocity I could muster, I said to my body, "Enough!" And amazingly—it listened! Within a week my temperature was almost normal, the symptoms were disappearing, and my weight was tipping the scale at close to 100 pounds.

Then followed a three-week period of different symptoms—mild symptoms that seemed to mirror what I experienced during chemo and radiation—the same rashes, the same mouth sores, and loss of my natural hair color for a few weeks of growth—exactly what happened before. Dr. Cursio was overjoyed. He explained this was the end of the clean-out, when the body retraces and dumps the residue of past toxicity that had slowly been worked out of the cells. Many times, as these substances move through the body on their way out, similar symptoms reappear that occurred the first time, but on a smaller scale.

Slowly my strength began to return and my weight increased. I was growing a new body. My hair was shinier, my nails were stronger, and I noticed old minor physical problems that had plagued me for years were suddenly clearing up. My skin, for instance, became totally clear after fifteen years of constant breakouts. And my menstrual cycle, which had completely stopped during the previous few months, now became regular for the first time in my life. The winter was over, spring was in the air, and I was blossoming. I deeply appreciated being alive.

In looking at the bigger picture—the first six months on my healing protocol, after I had finished conventional treatment, may have been about just stopping or even eradicating the cancer—but much of the underlying causes had yet to really be touched. I wasn't about to get off that easily. So the dues were paid, and the stuff of the chthonic realm, the blood and guts, worked its way out in order for deep healing to truly occur. And, I was very fortunate, indeed, that this transformative process had the protective and caring container of Joya's community in which to unfold.

Shortly after this period of time Dr. Cursio stopped coming to Florida on his usual monthly trips. He went into retirement and contact began to fade. I had gone through so much with him as my guide and support that it was sad and a little frightening to not have him there anymore. Still, I felt I had absorbed a lot of knowledge about how to care for myself and recognize different aspects of the healing process to now try and go it on my own.

9

Another Challenge

RECOVERING MY ENERGY AND STRENGTH WAS slow, very slow—baby steps at first. Even getting a massage was exhausting, since the cleaning and healing processes are being stimulated and that uses energy. At one point I decided to restart my yoga practice, and as I was doing a twist, I coughed, and up came a glob of blood. I called my oncologist in New York to find out if this was a radiation-related occurrence. He confided seeing instances where radiation scaring can harden tissue, making it easier to tear a capillary. He suggested a watch-and-wait approach. It happened only once more, and never again.

During this time, another ranch inhabitant, Billy, provided a new direction. Shortly after I was first diagnosed with lymphoma, Billy had been diagnosed with leukemia. He also followed Dr. Cursio's program and for several years remained symptom-free. But within the previous few months, Billy's spleen began to enlarge —a potentially dangerous symptom of leukemia. After much research he decided to try a healing modality called "The Kelly Program," which was being used at an alternative health clinic in Mexico. After a month at this clinic, his spleen was a normal size again. The Kelly Program incorporated a large amount of supplements, with wheatgrass juice and coffee enemas. It sounded cumbersome, but I was so impressed with Billy's results that I decided to try the program myself, thinking it might speed up recovery and increase my stamina.

The Kelly Program advised individual diet and supplementation based on an in-depth questionnaire and blood work results. The food program that was suggested for me was actually close to what I was already doing, so I pretty much kept my Cursio program intact. The supplements recommended were such a humongous amount, about 30 per meal, that by the time I swallowed half of them my stomach was already full. After two weeks, I was overwhelmed and simply couldn't take another pill.

The wheatgrass juice was interesting-tasting at first, with a strange sweet aftertaste, but after two weeks I developed such a tremendous repulsion towards it that even just thinking about the smell made me sick to my stomach. My body rebelled and ended that.

The last part of the program was the coffee enemas, which were surprisingly not too unpleasant. Coffee is supposed to stimulate the action of the liver to release toxins and force a cleansing of sorts. A by-product of administering coffee rectally was a mildly intoxicating feeling, which I didn't mind one bit. I did though have some doubts about the possible negative side effects of continually washing out the colon and over-stimulating the liver, but decided to try this anyway.

Four weeks into the coffee enema routine, I awoke one morning with pains in my chest and down my arms, especially when I took a deep breath. Considering the variety of symptoms I had experienced during the previous months, I thought perhaps this was just another cleansing, and was not alarmed. I simply rested for a few days. On the fourth morning, as I bent down to pick something up, my heart seemed to "pop" and then go haywire—beating erratically and speeding up to over 200 beats per minute. I immediately lay down and tried to relax, but after 15 minutes with no let-up, I felt as though I was going to pass out. I quickly called a friend, a nurse, who lived on the ranch. Upon seeing me she insisted I be rushed to the hospital. In Emergency I was hooked up to several machines that monitored my heart and was given valium. Gradually my heartbeat began to slow down, and after four hours it was back to normal.

I was kept in the hospital for testing, and it appeared I had an enlarged heart and excess fluid in my chest cavity. In the X-rays, the left side of my chest was so covered with scar tissue that it was difficult to see clearly what was going on. After a few days of calm I decided to make use of the hospital's services and make my stay as comfortable as possible. I requested a waterbed mattress and a physical therapy massage. After the massage I sat in a hot tub with jets pulsating all around me. One particular jet was positioned precisely in a way that caused a heightened sexual reaction—and off my heart went, back into an erratic wild heartbeat. I quickly got out of the tub and then proceeded to vomit. The doctors became alarmed and immediately admitted me to intensive care. In the end, I was too embarrassed to tell the true cause of this latest escapade. After a few hours, fortunately, my heart again slowed down. By this time, the doctors were so perplexed by my case and due to the complexity of my health history, they suggested I be sent back to New York Hospital to be treated by my original doctor.

Waiting for me at the entrance of New York Hospital was my oncologist, who ushered me into a small treatment cubicle. After a quick five-minute exam, he felt that the cancer probably had returned, but alas—now there were new chemotherapy drugs available. He also mentioned I might need open chest surgery to release the fluid around my heart. And this was all before I even checked in!

During the next few days, being in a teaching hospital, several doctors came around to check on me and evaluate my symptoms. Most of their reactions to my health regimen over the last three years were extremely negative. They felt it was terribly irresponsible of me not to get proper medical care for my previous health crisis—although my own doctor later confessed that the illness and recovery didn't follow any medical guidelines he knew of. The doctors thought my whole idea of a healing crisis was folly, and I started to find my faith being shaken by this onslaught of criticism. In Florida, I had solid support from Joya and my friends to help me through shaky times, but here in New York, I felt alone and cut off, and bombarded by a harsh medical world filled with machines, needles and fear.

I started to doubt the importance of my last three years on the diet, but when I realized that nothing had been proven yet, that I was still alive, and my beliefs were the only things I had to hold on to, suddenly I held on tight. Within me a powerful urgency to get well once again began to arise, and again I started to do intense healing meditations each night. The only comforting element was the presence of my dear mother, who tirelessly helped maintain my food regimen—even carting a juicer to the hospital. The hospital staff was not at all pleased, but upon my mother's insistence, they allowed her the space to carry on.

The first time I was in the hospital everything was new and I was curious, but this time, it was like cold steel. I saw it with different eyes. While there I met two other people my age with lymphoma. I was witness to the devastating effects of the "new" treatments, which for one of them wasn't even working.

I was put through many kinds of tests, some of which I refused, feeling they were too toxic or dangerous. The decisive test was a CT scan, something that was not yet available three years before when I was first in the hospital. Lying next to me in the prep room, waiting for my turn on the CT machine at 11:30 pm at night, was a comatose woman. She was completely white like a ghost, and hooked up to several IV's. I was so shaken by her condition that I sat there, doing my visualization work with scalding intensity, and hung tight to the possibility of my symptoms being just another healing crisis.

After six days in the hospital, my oncologist entered my room with final test results and a big smile. According to the scan, my heart was back to normal size, the excess fluid in my chest cavity was gone and, as far as they could tell, there was no cancer present, period!

"NO CANCER PRESENT!!!!" Over three years of living with the discomfort of "not-knowing" and now to hear these words—incredible! Something worked! Everything worked—all the guidance, all the effort, all the nudges, prayers, reminders, and so much grace.

It actually took me a few weeks to fully let those words in. My diagnosis changed to pericarditis, an inflammation of the lining of the heart—something common in people who had radiation in that area. Rest was all the treatment required as the inflammation appeared to be almost resolved by itself.

Leaving the hospital was much different than three years earlier, when I was still enveloped in a naive protective bubble. This time I sobbed—for the horror of what could have been and was for the others still there—and for the precious fragile gift of freedom to move on in my life.

10

Fine Tuning

*A*FTER RECOVERING FROM PERICARDITIS, MY energy and strength returned and my sense of wellness continued to expand. Every few months though for the next few years, other lesser cleansing/healing episodes would emerge as the underground work was still resolving.

One cleansing process involved aches and pains in lymph nodes around my body, espescially behind my ears and neck—something that happened a lot as a teenager. The nodes became sore and swelled for a few days, then would go back down, only to swell again a week later. At the same time I also awoke each morning feeling as though I had an extreme hangover. Sometimes it would take until two in the afternoon before I could focus properly. These symptoms continued for about five weeks, each time becoming a little more intense until they reached a pitch that was becoming difficult to handle. And then suddenly, one morning, all of the symptoms were completely gone.

Another episode started with a bad cold, coughing up large amounts of yellow thick mucus. Of course colds are connected to viruses, but Dr. Cursio would say that the gift of a cold is that it amplifies cleansing actions in the upper respiratory area, pushing out any waste and clearing any build-up of debris. The cold lasted about two weeks, yet I continued to cough up large amounts of thick yellow mucus. After three months with no let-up, Dr. Harry became alarmed that I had a chest infection and strongly suggested I take antibiotics. To me, this was just another detoxification (and not a serious one at that), especially since, except for the cough, I felt fine. But in a moment of weakness and carelessness, I consented to take the medication, just to get over the discomfort more quickly. I figured that I could cleanse any remaining waste from my lungs another time—after I had a break.

I took the full course of strong antibiotics, and after two weeks nothing changed—the mucus was still there as before, though the medicine did cause quite a reaction elsewhere. I developed an itchy rash on my behind that after a few days turned into open blisters. A week later I developed a raging yeast infection, for which Dr.

Harry prescribed anti-yeast medication, but to no avail. After the third anti-yeast medication failed, and with the discomfort becoming more intense, it was time to get creative. I found some temporary solutions to the yeast problem, having to do with yogurt and other things, but when I stopped their use the symptoms returned.

Finally I reached a point of desperation. I stopped and looked more closely at these challenges, and slowly ideas began to form. I remembered back when I had developed my first yeast infection in my teens—after a round of antibiotics—and had been given a suppository, which wasn't even prescribed anymore due to all the new broad-spectrum medicines now on the market. I asked Dr. Harry for a prescription for two weeks-worth of the old tablets, though he tried to dissuade me, thinking they were old school and didn't really work very well. But at my insistence, he gave in.

I also remembered, years back, reading an article about the connection between high blood sugar and yeast infections. I was consuming 2 pounds of fruit and 12 ounces of carrot juice daily, which contained a lot of natural sugar, and I suspected that this high sugar intake could be a contributing factor in feeding my problem. Therefore I decided to stop eating fruit and changed to tomato and celery juice while I was doing my new intensive approach. I also read from a few different sources that high vitamin B complex could be helpful with clearing yeast infections, so I began taking 150 mg daily for the duration of my new treatment protocol.

The final contributing factor was doing healing visualizations and prayer—every day, three times a day.

After two weeks on my self-wrought program, much to my great relief, the yeast infection was gone! At the same time, the idea popped into my mind to try using vitamin E oil on the sores on my behind. I'd cut open a capsule and rub the oil into the inflamed areas a few times a day. After three days the sores were all healed, but as soon as I stopped applying the oil they returned, so I repeated the treatment. After three episodes, they were totally gone—for good!

I had been an artist most of my life and so appreciated being able to turn my creative focus on figuring out how to successfully resolve these challenges. It was not only a huge relief, but at the same time the discovery of new healing supports was exciting!

As for coughing up mucus, that continued for a full year, and then one day it was gone—and I didn't catch another cold for six years—until I spent time in Los Angeles smog.

After that, my strength increased and I was able to exert more physical energy than I had in the previous few years, doing yoga, hiking and swimming.

With all of this new-found exercise, I started to become aware of a slight ache in the back of my left hip. When I had been in the hospital two years before with pericarditis, one of the tests I underwent was a bone marrow extraction from the back of my left hip, which in itself was not painful, yet left me with a slight pinching feeling that would occur sporadically. But now that feeling was intensifying and I was becoming concerned. I was treated by a chiropractor a few times, but to no avail. Then a few weeks later as I reached to pick up a large plant, the muscles in my lower back went into spasm and I was flat on my back for three days. After that I was able to move around, but only with a fair amount of pain, especially in the left hip area where I'd had the bone marrow taken. Then after another two weeks of hobbling around, I started to feel ill—weak, with loss of appetite, colorless and achy. On the second day, the pain in my hip increased drastically to the point where I could barely walk. On the third day I awoke, and to my amazement, I was fully recovered—the pain and all other symptoms were completely resolved.

11

Moving On

*I*N READING THESE ACCOUNTS OF MY EXPERI-
ences, one may wonder how I managed emotionally
and psychologically during the various crises—how I
had the faith that I was healing instead of dying of cancer or seriously ill with something else. The truth is
that I was never sure. There were many occasions
when I had strong doubts and fears to contend with,
especially after Dr. Cursio was no longer available to
consult with, and without another substitute support
system that came close.

Many times I felt a tug of war between viewing my
situation positively or negatively. A voice would creep
into my head questioning if I were crazy and naïve to
believe such symptoms could truly be a healing

process. I would deal with this by breathing slowly, relaxing my muscles and attempting to hold an awareness of simply "not knowing." Reminding myself, repeatedly, that I truly did not know the outcome kept me from becoming either overly optimistic or pessimistic. It helped me to be present, rather than jumping into the future. I was able to find calm solace in the "not knowing" present moment.

I also felt compelled at times to consider the medical route, which I occasionally did, taking various tests like blood work or X-rays, just to get more information on what my symptoms were about. Most of the time, the results were reassuring, though sometimes they were inconclusive, leaving my medical doctors scratching their heads about the mysteriousness of my symptoms, their progression and ultimately, their resolution.

During the years since then, I've continued to go through healing episodes that have manifested in almost every part of my body at one time or another — literally from my hair to my toes. Whatever form it comes in, I can always feel the energy drain from my muscles as it is directed inwards towards the area that needs to be addressed. I seem to naturally lose my appetite and prefer vegetable juices or blended vegetable soups, plus lots of rest. And it passes, and my appetite comes back strong, and I usually feel a surge of new energy.

These episodes are much less frequent now and usually subtler, to the degree that I actually feel healthier now than I can ever remember feeling. My energy is good, my digestion is fine, my hormones are in balance, and no aches or pains or complaints. The Chinese have a saying, "Health is the silence of the organs." I can attest to that!

By 1981, after six years of living in Joya's community, I knew it was time to leave. I left with an open heart and deep, deep appreciation for so many things — especially in regards to my healing. I'm not sure I would have been able to get through it all without their support, and without Joya's special care.

I settled in California, and almost immediately started receiving phone calls from people in health crises, wanting information about what I had done to heal. I shared my story many times over, and gave pointers as best I could, especially since Dr. Cursio was retired. This book emerged from that time as I felt myself pulled more and more towards supporting others in their healing journey. Eventually I saw the writing on the wall, and fully stepped into the health care field, going back to school for my degree in nutrition. To complete my education and gain experience, I then apprenticed with another health care practitioner who was closer to my view of nutrition and healing than traditional dietitians.

I was to see Dr. Cursio one last time a few years later in New York. I called him to say hello and was able to meet for a little while. When I walked into his apartment we just smiled at each other and laughed. (The last time he had seen me was four years before in the grips of my major detoxification, weighing 90 pounds and looking like a ghost.) He took my hand and said, "You must really have a powerful will to live. You know, don't you, that it was more than just the diet?" Considering how food-oriented he was, I was a little shocked to hear these words! I paused for a moment, then replied, "Yes, I do know. Yet I believe my 'will to live' led me to you and gave me the focus and committment to follow your wise counsel to the best of my ability. And for that, I will always be grateful."

Section Two: Healing Resources

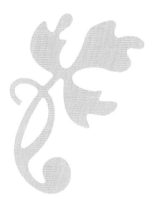

12

A Common-Sense Approach to Healing and Disease

*W*HETHER YOU NOW HAVE CANCER OR HAVE been treated with chemotherapy, radiation or surgery, the threat of it growing back and metastasizing is greater if the conditions that allowed it to grow in the first place are not changed or addressed. The problem with traditional medical treatment is that, at the cost of potentially severe physical damage to the body, usually only the malignancy is treated and not the underlying cause.

In attempting to understand the underlying cause, it is important to look more closely at why both adults and children are developing cancer and other degenerative diseases such as arthritis, heart disease, and diabetes at increasingly alarming rates. These are not diseases of germs. On the physical* level, they are diseases of bodily pollution, imbalance, and/or insufficient nutrient intake. More than ever before, science is recognizing the connection between poor diets, stress, chemicals in our environment, and many common disorders.

In order to stop and reverse the degenerative processes, whether it be arresting cancer or clearing plaque from arteries, we must first accept a great amount of the responsibility for what occurs to us in disease, in healing, and in health—whether it is food choices, ignoring the need to protect against toxic environments, or stress. It is crucial to understand the influences that undermine our health as well as the influences that encourage healing and preserve health —on all levels, and then act upon this information wholeheartedly to bring about a true transformation.

The body has in it the knowledge and ability to heal itself, more profoundly than most people realize, even in some extreme cases with cancer, provided there is still enough vital energy available to carry out the work. The key to bringing this innate healing force into action is, first, by removing all obstructing, irritating, or

---

*Footnote: (I differentiate here between physical influences and influences on the emotional, psychological and spiritual levels. I believe disease can be rooted on different levels, in varying degrees with each individual.)

hindering influences. Then, through a high-nutrient wholesome diet, focused attitude, and healthful lifestyle, one can create the optimum conditions for both a physiological and a psychological environment where healing action can operate more fully. That this process actually works is not a great mystery—it is a basic law of cause and effect.

It sounds almost too simple but the difficulty lies, not in just recognizing the body's needs, but in the actual breaking of old established unhealthful habits and, even more so, in allowing the cleansing and healing crises that do occur to run their natural course.

When supporting the healing process, one cannot expect a lifetime of stored waste, toxins, unhealthy tissue or sluggish organs to simply clear with a good diet and healthful way of living. The body needs to clean out, repair and rebuild. For some people this process is barely perceptible as most of the deep reparative work occurs during sleep when the body has the most use of its energy. But sometimes, especially in my case, cleansing and repair symptoms spill into waking hours, and this can cause a degree of discomfort and fear. Millions of dollars are spent each year on relieving these discomforts by drugs that can suppress the symptoms, and therefore keep the impurities in the body that otherwise would have been excreted. Thus the body is kept from doing its cleansing work, and on top of that, chemicals, which cannot be utilized by the body in any nourishing way, are now added to the original waste. If this process is repeated until the body is overloaded with impurities, it will become sluggish and toxic, and more serious illness will occur. This usually happens in the weakest spot of the body, where the most toxic material has accumulated.

As for addressing the emotional, psychological and spiritual influences, certainly seeking out helpful support—through therapists, books, and practices such as yoga and meditation—can help shift perception, enabling greater clarity and a release of old negative patterns. And work on one level can pour into other layers. Taking the time and care to prepare and consume wholesome foods, for instance, and the willingness to struggle with and give up old unhealthful habits is a deep message of love to ourselves. And that message of self-love may ultimately be the elixir that empowers us to heal on many levels, to the greatest degree we are capable of.

13

Attitude in the Healing Process

*F*ROM THE BEGINNING OF THIS BOOK I HAVE attempted to emphasize the great importance of attitude in healing. When I first was piecing together my healing container I came across a line in a book that cut deep. It was that most ordinary people take everything that happens to them in life either as a blessing or a curse, whereas a warrior takes everything that happens as a challenge. I knew in that moment, to survive I needed to become a warrior.

I've come to appreciate, in dealing with disease or disasters of any kind, in order to best meet the challenges of life one must become a kind of warrior. Laziness and mediocrity have no place here. It is crucial that the mind become concentrated and focused, and intuition valued.

I believe strongly that for every person there is choice—there are clues, pointers, and guidance available. If you have the powerful determination to search, ask, invite, petition, even if there is tremendous fear and doubt, despite all obstacles, you will find relevant information and inspiration, and that which is truly needed. Of course, what we truly need depends on our staging in life (not necessarily our age). Once one becomes sensitive to it, it is shocking how much life continually offers healing possibilities. Yet at some point with all of us, what we need may be about how to let go of life—with dignity, ease and trust, if possible. The point is to become in touch with the unfolding, and to somehow place ourselves in alignment with it, which means to open and to work with it as best we can to the fullest degree possible.

In difficult situations, health and otherwise, I have found ritual to be powerful and gifting. I light a candle symbolic of lighting the way. I ask for what I need for healing or resolution, calling forth help and guidance from Spirit, from the Masters, from ancestors, from supportive friends and family. Afterwards, I feel it is important to be aware of, and to be open and sensitive to messages that can come from opening a book, from a conversation, from a dream. Information and guidance will come—it's just a matter of recognizing it—and one will, if closer attention is paid to what we hear, see, feel or intuit.

Many times though, with a cancer diagnosis people feel overwhelmed, powerless, riddled with fear, and desperate to find distraction—wanting to get away from the intensity and fright. Friends and family may think they are helping by supporting distractions—helping to get away from the issue at hand. There is a fine line between being a soothing influence and loving support, as opposed to helping dilute the focus that may be needed.

And, as I suggested earlier in the book, fear can serve. It can rip a person out of "everyday" reality and give them the capacity to focus, deepen, and act—way beyond what they normally would do or even could do. We may not be able to erase the fear, but we can choose what we do with it. We can feel the fear, and detach enough to recognize its intensity and power and then make use of it to motivate us. On the other hand, fear can freeze people, weaken their resolve, and cloud their wisdom. Supporting people to make use of this powerful force can be of huge help.

The challenge to get involved and work with the healing process can sometimes start out seeming enormously difficult and overwhelming. Yet, when one is willing, the effort itself can transform not only the physical condition, but also our character and state of awareness. And, it can expand our wisdom, experience and understanding of this mystery we call "life."

14

The Power of Visualization

*W*HILE IN THE HOSPITAL THE FIRST TIME, A friend sent me a cassette tape called "Imagery Meditation in the Healing of Cancer" by Dr. O. Carl Simonton. He was an oncologist who had suggested to a few of his terminally ill patients to visualize their cancer becoming smaller and disappearing—and amazingly so, some completely healed. He then became a full-time pioneer in teaching people to tap into the power of their minds, or imagination, or whatever part of our beings respond to imagining a healing scenario.

Even before that I remember watching a segment of the TV news show, *60 Minutes*, reporting on a similar thing. A practitioner was directing a woman to visualize the disappearance of a large mole on the back of her neck. After one month it was completely gone. It was one of those memories I never forgot.

It is said that we only use about 5 percent of our brains. What potential lies in the other 95 percent? I wholeheartedly believe the ability to create healing changes through concentrated intention is one of them, and the time is ripe for this new potential to manifest as a useable resource to influence change in our lives. For those of us who have tapped into this resource, through concentration and visualization, not just with our thoughts but with images, feelings, smells—all the sensate stimulation we can muster— plus inviting divine intervention or the mystery that is in all healing—anything is possible—and there are many of us alive to verify it.

The moments spent in visualizing my own body healing nourished me in a potent way. It felt as though prayer was made more tangible—helping myself while asking for help. It connected me more deeply to my own healing process. It helped calm my mind and ease my fears. At those times when my fears were strongly engaged, my visualization felt empowered and even more intense and one-pointed. I quickly discovered that was a great use of fear—to put it into visualization!

I highly recommend visualization before operations or treatment—imagining what one wants to see transpire.

As far as subject matter on what to visualize—it's an

open field. Personally, I think the more creative, the better. The actions to bring about change can range from waging war to transforming with a kiss. There are many CDs available as well as individual therapists who walk the listener through different imagery—making it easier to get started until one can connect with what is most relevant.

A friend of mine, while undergoing chemotherapy, at the beginning of each treatment would bless and welcome the chemotherapy agents and request of the drugs to bless him with their wisdom to discriminate between those cells that needed to die and those that needed to remain strong, healthy and protected. He then wore headphones playing dramatic heart-centered music that helped him visualize images and feelings of energy swirling and finding its way to the tumor as the "healing" work was being done. His results after the chemo sessions were astounding. Not only was there an unusually rapid reduction of the tumor, but he also had very few side effects with otherwise extremely toxic infusions.

Besides using visualization as a healing resource, it can also be a powerful tool for influencing and creating what we need and aspire to in all other facets of life.

15

Dream Work

*W*HEN IN A CRISIS, HEALTH OR OTHERWISE, dreams can be a rich source of guidance that spring to the forefront. They certainly have been a powerful part of my healing process—from the first dream with Sai Baba that inferred there was a problem inside my chest, two years before I was diagnosed. After that, many of my dreams gave reassuring feedback suggesting I was on a healing path, while others alerted me to things I was ignoring and needed to pay more attention to.

Most of these dreams were not obvious in their meaning at first, but after rereading them over a period of time, I could see the similarities with what was happening in my life, and had a felt-sense of connection between my dreams and health challenges.

I so deeply appreciate dreams as precious gifts! I feel they are the communication between our waking consciousness with all its desires, fears and judgments, and the deeper knowing part of ourselves that is free of superficial conditioning. Dreams come in many forms and serve many functions—from helping to release stress, to being a guiding light. Even if we don't remember them, they may still provide their support. But if we do remember them, we are presented with an opportunity to gain insight, guidance and healing.

Dreams occur usually in the same language that we ordinarily use, but in actuality, they also speak a different language—a language of symbols, myths and archetypes that have developed slowly since the beginning of human existence, and perhaps, even before. An example is the symbol of the sun. Throughout history, the sun has come to symbolize the Great Father, the inner light of awareness, a healing presence, and so on.

There are stories after stories—from the Bible and many other sources—that have described how dreams accurately predicted future occurrences as well as gave amazing information, especially regarding scientific breakthroughs, and even providing complete healing.

The practice of dream interpretation is a vast field with many gifted dream tenders, yet interpreting dreams can be experienced by anyone with the willingness, patience and open-mindedness to spend time with the dream and ask themselves some relevant questions. For instance, how do each of the dream characters represent different parts of myself? Is the main challenge in the dream something that is familiar with anything going on in my life or similar to a common fairytale or myth? Does each object or symbol in the dream stir memories or reactions or remind me about something? At some point in working with the dream there is usually a felt sense or "ah ha!"—clues to what is alive in the meaning. Dreams are multi-layered and could not only be about something personal, but also something collective—about the world in general. As I reread old dreams, I find the meaning deepens and sometimes even changes. And although there are no absolutes when it comes to dream interpretation, just attempting to get out of it what stirs may be of benefit.

In serious health crises, if dreams come forth and are clearly remembered, I strongly encourage people to write them down and connect with a psychologist or other person who works with dreams, or a dream circle— a group of people who work on each other's dreams. It is also possible to petition help through a dream by simply asking, before going to sleep, to be gifted with a guide dream in regard to a specific situation. Keep a pen and paper next to your bed—and within a few nights, if not right away, something usually comes.

16

Nutritional Program

*D*R. CURSIO ADVISED ME ON THE FOLLOWING food regimen with slight variations every month. He stressed the importance of eating the full quantity of food prescribed, and to eat the food in the specific order he suggested.

His programs for most people were basically the same format, but each person had something a little different for their specific constitution and current challenges. Dr. Cursio used iridology to determine those needs.

Each meal began with a freshly prepared vegetable juice, followed with a salad put through a blender to pre-digest it. These foods were in a form rapidly absorbed by the body, with minimal digestive energy used. Next was a more complex food—fruit for breakfast and lunch, and steamed vegetables for dinner. This would be followed by the most concentrated and complex foods —either nuts or eggs for breakfast, nuts or occasionally goat cheese for lunch, and potatoes, whole grains, beans or yams for dinner.

Eating according to this food system allows the body to quickly break down simple foods first, and then progress to levels of increasing complexity—all to insure the most efficient and least wasteful use of digestive energy. Conserving energy along with abundant nutrients are the "KEY" to empowering the body's own pre-programmed natural healing capacities to operate at full potency. This supports the cells to do the best cleansing, repair and regenerative work they are capable of.

Throughout the years I have come to appreciate that Dr. Cursio's programs are among the simplest yet most potent activator of the cleansing and healing process. They are not about forcing the body to cleanse by consuming non-food substances, such as clays and Epsom salts or using intense saunas. Instead, the body is deeply, deeply nourished and is able to gather its forces when it is ready, and then mount cleansing and repair actions that are more profound and able to go deeper than any manipulative, forced cleansing can go.

Dr. Cursio's Food Program
as prescribed for Dale Figtree

Breakfast
- 8 oz of fresh vegetable juice—half carrot and half celery
- 12 oz of blended salad—consisting of 4 leaves of romaine or red leaf lettuce, 1 tomato, ½ red bell pepper, ½ cucumber, ½ lemon—put in blender and blended until semi-liquid
- 1 lb of apples
- 1 oz of raw almonds (occasionally this was changed to 1 soft-boiled egg or 1 oz of sesame butter)

Lunch
- 8 oz of the same vegetable juice
- 16 oz of blended salad
- 1 lb of fresh fruit (seasonal and only one variety each day)
- 4 oz of raw nuts (almonds twice a week, filberts twice a week, walnuts, pecans, raw peanuts, sunflower seeds, pumpkin seeds)

Occasionally, instead of nuts, 4 oz of raw goat cheese was added.

Dinner
- 8 oz of the same vegetable juice
- 16 oz of blended salad
- 1 lb of two steamed vegetables (different colors)
- A complex carbohydrate or concentrated protein food—each night different

For example: One night—1 lb yams; another night—1 lb potatoes. Other nights were 4 oz lentils, lima beans or other beans (dry weight before cooked), or 4 oz brown rice, millet or other whole grain (dry weight before cooked)

Snacks
Popcorn, rice cakes, raw vegetable sticks, and herb teas
Oil: cold-pressed olive oil in glass
Spices allowed
No salt or soy

For my specific program, Dr. Cursio advised 1 lb of yams at least three or four nights a week. Rarely did he give yams to other people more than once or twice a week.

Dr. Cursio usually advised me to put carrots in my juice, whereas most other people would get carrots in their juice only occasionally, being prescribed instead tomato/cucumber/ celery juice.

Eggs needed to be organically raised and cooked in boiling water for 4 minutes.

Potatoes and yams were to be steamed, as were all the vegetables—no sautéing. Vegetables were to be cooked whole when possible, as this preserves most of the vitamins.

Twice a month Dr. Cursio gave most people, including me, banana dinners consisting of:
- 8 oz of vegetable juice,
- 16 oz of blended salad
- 4 ripe bananas

Otherwise, bananas and coconuts were not to be eaten in place of fruit.

All water, especially for cooking grains and steaming vegetables, needed to be distilled—including drinking water.

Salad dressing usually was composed of lemon juice and olive oil.

Popcorn, as a snack, needed to be air-popped. Olive oil, kelp powder, and yeast flakes could be sprinkled on top.

My personal experience with the food program went through a few phases. It was a new challenge and an exciting adventure. I liked all the food, but the quantities took getting used to. At first it took hours to finish dinner, but after three weeks my body was sucking up the food like a sponge.

After about two months, resistance started to flare along with cravings for junk food and meat products that I hadn't eaten or wanted in years. I went through a stage of hating blended salads and hating cleaning the juicer, and even more so, resented people who could eat Big Macs and hot dogs. At times I became jealous, angry and frustrated; still I felt my life was at stake so I managed to resist temptation and not cheat. Soon the resistance lost power and faded away, and I began to appreciate simple tastes more than ever before. Through my experience and others, I've come to understand it is a three-phase process most people go through when changing long-term habits. First there is the honeymoon stage, and second, the discontentment, when old habits try to regain control—sometimes with a vengeance. And then the ease of the third stage, when the changes become "normal" and appreciated.

Through the months and years, I go back and forth between loving the program and feeling other cravings. I've learned to create more interesting recipes, which helps to fulfill my occasional desire for something fancier. Yet, after all this time, the food program is no longer a food program for me, but a way of life, and the simple beauty of it is something I truly enjoy and appreciate.

After five years on the Cursio diet I came across a book by Dr. Harold Mannors called *The Death of Cancer*. Dr. Mannors was chairman of the biology department at Loyola University in Chicago. He was working on a research project involving laetrile, which was the subject of his book. In his experiments on mice with malignant tumors, he found by administering laetrile alone, the results were not remarkable. But by combining laetrile with high doses of vitamin A and protein digestive enzymes, the results were startling. With one particular type of breast tumor, he had an 89 percent cure rate. Through his research, he came to believe the action of the vitamin A and the enzymes served to weaken and break down the outer coating of the cancer cell, allowing the laetrile to easily enter and interact with the cell, releasing its poison and thereby killing the cell. This interaction does not occur with a healthy cell, only with malignant types.

In relating this information to the food program that Dr. Cursio prescribed for me, the carrot juice I drank three times a day and the yams three or four times a week supplied huge quantities of vitamin A.

The raw salads and raw nuts supplied a rich source of digestive enzymes, and the almonds and yams are known to contain a newly discovered and controversial vitamin, B 17, which is laetrile in its natural state. Out of all the other food programs Dr. Cursio prescribed, mine always had the largest quantity of these particular foods.

Note

For people considering embarking upon this food program or a similar approach, I cannot emphasize enough the importance of seeking out a nutritional health counselor who is knowledgeable about the cleansing and healing processes that will occur—a person who can guide you and advise special dietary changes to help these processes complete themselves without complications. Detoxification is not difficult to understand intellectually, yet when a healing action actually happens, without a good support system, most people panic. Once a depth of cleansing is opened, it doesn't necessarily close back down without some kind of resistance. After all, the body's intelligence knows what would ultimately be the best for its health and longevity, and once it connects to that, it does not want to let go until the work is complete.

17

Detoxification and the Healing Process

*I*T WAS DIFFICULT FOR ME TO BELIEVE AT FIRST that acute illnesses could actually lead to better health, especially growing up viewing "being sick" as something to fear and to fight. But after a few months under Dr. Cursio's care, I started to understand acute symptoms as detoxification actions that carried impurities out of the body. Recognizing this enabled me to accept most of these episodes with less fear and resistance.

By looking more deeply at the symptoms of most acute illnesses such as colds and flu, it starts to become obvious how material is being eliminated, usually by amplifying the body's own natural actions. Even though germs or viruses may be the initial cause, they also serve as a form of "spring cleaning" that can clear the build-up of waste in the body. The cells produce mucus in response to an invasion or irritation, and that mucus not only carries out the "germs" or irritants, but also carries out accumulated waste and debris along the way. This may be why people in cities and areas of air pollution tend to get more colds and upper respiratory infections. The irony is that these acute illnesses can be a cleansing and restorative gift.

Some common cleansing actions are: sweats, headaches, skin breakouts and rashes, fever, coughs, painful swollen lymph glands, mouth ulcers, excess mucus and other discharges, and intestinal upsets, especially loose stools and vomiting. Along with these can come symptoms of tiredness, gas, unpleasant breath, rapid pulse, achiness, sensitive teeth, stiff joints, yellowish skin, pains in the feet, back, and major organs, shortness of breath, muscle weakness, and depression.

As the body cleans itself out of old stored-up toxic material and replaces diseased or damaged tissue, a process called retracing or reversal can occur. This happens when toxic substances that have been stored in the organs or muscles of the body begin to be released and eliminated from the system. As they are carried out of the body, they usually pass through the bloodstream, kidneys, intestines, skin, lungs or lymph system. During this journey, the toxins or waste some-times cause reactions due to their poisonous or irritat-ing nature. These reactions are usually the same as the symptoms when the original problem first occurred. Old diseases, drugs or physical problems are sometimes re-experienced, usually on a smaller scale for a short time. Then, as the toxic material or diseased tissue finally leaves the body, that bit of history is gone once and for all. Sometimes the symptoms are so obviously the same as a previous challenge or medication, even from decades before, it is downright uncanny!

Dr. Cursio felt that we need not worry about com-plications if we take care of our body when early symp-toms of a cleansing action appear. I have witnessed this many times, not only with myself, but with several peo-ple at the ranch, who while doing the food program developed symptoms that I never imagined would be possible to heal without medical intervention. They experienced things like boils, fevers, extreme rashes, styes, infections of many kinds, and an assortment of other ailments. Extreme conditions were usually not just left alone to heal by themselves. Under Dr. Cursio's instructions, there were many supportive resources to employ that did not suppress symptoms, but that would encourage them to cleanse more quick-ly. An example is, for boils, applying flax seed poul-tices—flax seeds heated with water to make a gel and then applied to a boil to draw pus more quickly to the surface. There were many tricks in Dr. Cursio's healing bag.

Dr. Cursio would constantly emphasize that during a detoxification process, it was essential to support the cleansing and repair action by reducing energy demands on all levels. Therefore more energy was available to be used by the body to go to the depths of what was needed for the healing work.

Reducing energy demands means rest—physically, emotionally and mentally. On the physical level it means reducing activity and sleeping—as much as possible. While sleeping, all reparative and recuperative processes are freer to operate with greater potency, since more energy is available.

During these occurrences, it is important to keep warm, so energy is not compromised and pulled to the surface to maintain body temperature.

Digestive rest is also of utmost importance during a detox process, since a big chunk of energy is used in the digestive, absorptive and assimilation processes. When the actions of intensified cleansing and repair are present, the appetite usually reduces naturally so that the body's energy is able to remain in the area where the deeper work is occurring. During these times, Dr. Cursio advised refraining from eating solid food and instead suggested either vegetable juices, or blended vegetable soups or just distilled water— depending on the severity of the symptoms and the person's general constitution.

The juices consisted of an 8 oz freshly made vegetable juice—usually a combination of one tomato and the rest, celery and cucumber. Three hours later this would be followed by 8 oz of freshly made fruit juice (one variety only). These juices were to be alternated throughout the day. In this form, the nutrients could be absorbed very quickly with little digestive energy demand, so less energy would be pulled away from the area being focused on. When symptoms of the detox resolved, the change to a normal diet would be gradual—just juices, salads and fruit first, or blended vegetable soups. Then after a day or so, the full program could be resumed.

Resting and conserving energy during cleansing and repair symptoms includes avoiding conditions that use up energy unnecessarily. When bathing, for instance, the temperature of the water should not be very hot, as this causes the body to speed up its respiration in an effort to maintain normal body temperature, and is an unnecessary waste of energy. This is one of the reasons for feeling limp and tired after a hot bath or shower—a good deal of energy has been expended.

The same holds true for sunbathing. A moderate exposure is necessary and even healing, but too much sun causes the heart to beat faster and the body to use its energy for cooling down, creating an unnecessary energy depletion.

18

Exercise

*B*ESIDES DIET, EXERCISE IS ANOTHER MAJOR component that supports health and balance. But when ill or experiencing detoxification symptoms, exercise can rob the body of precious vitality that would otherwise be used for cleansing and repair work.

When upgrading dietary changes, usually during the first few months energy is more concentrated interiorly, clearing out old stored waste and toxicity from the liver and other organs, as well as reversing degenerative conditions. Most people lose weight at this time, even though the calorie count of their food intake is plentiful. Dr. Cursio would remind us many times over that the initial weight loss is due to cleaning out old stuff. The very high nutrient intake actually stimulates the metabolism to function at a higher level, and the first thing the body wants to do when it has more raw materials and energy available is to take care of interior healing needs.

Therefore, when increasing nutrient intake, instead of pulling the extra resources straight into the muscles, which strong exercise demands, there is wisdom in reducing exercise for a time. This allows the extra raw materials and energy to be used as the body chooses to direct it. During this period, simple walking or very light exercise is all that should be done.

When and if cleansing and repair symptoms start to occur, it is most important to stop all unnecessary physical activity and rest as much as possible, so that the body's energy can be fully directed towards the area of the inner healing work. At these times energy is pulled from the outside to the inside, and people experience weakness or tiredness—just like with a flu or a cold. Once the cleansing, healing actions subside, the energy returns, usually a little stronger than before.

At some point in this process, which is different for each person, the energy is once again fully available to the muscles. The time is then ripe to jump back into an exercise program—hopefully that one truly enjoys—which challenges the muscles and heart in a way that builds strength and tone, rather than depletes.

19

Toxic vs. Non-Toxic

*T*HERE IS NO LONGER ANY DOUBT THAT THE chemicals released into our foods and environment have contributed greatly to a rapid increase in degenerative diseases, such as cancer, birth defects, arthritis, asthma, autoimmune disorders, and on and on. Chemicals can also affect brain chemistry, creating imbalances that may manifest as Attention Deficit Disorder (ADD), depression or anxiety. The bottom line is, how can we protect ourselves, our families and our communities from this insidious toxicity and damage, and also support and create higher health standards in industry and in our homes?

The main way to protect oneself is through education—discovering what is toxic and what alternatives exist. There are excellent books on the market and websites that discuss this relevant information. One of these books is *Home Safe Home* by Debra Dadd. For every product that has toxicity, there are alternative clean products to be found.

Categories where one needs to pay particular attention and read labels are:

Toxic chemicals in the food chain: Chemical additives in processed foods; pesticide residue on foods; hormone additives and antibiotics in farm animals; mercury in large fish; canola oil (one of 200 substances tested by the Susan Korman Cancer Foundation and found to contribute to breast cancer in lab animals), non-stick coated cookware; and plastic containers that water and food are stored and cooked in.

Buying or growing organically raised food, if possible, means more nutrients in the food. It also means no chemicals for the body to deal with and waste energy in defensive demands.

Household products: Detergents—for clothes, dishes, and dishwashers; softener sheets for the dryer; most household cleaners and disinfectants (especially those containing ammonia or bleach); oven cleaners; floor cleaners; furniture polishes; mildew removers; bug sprays; house paints and solvents; gasoline fumes; and car polishes.

Skin and hair products and make-up: The chemicals that we put on our bodies get absorbed! Most skin products have irritating or toxic chemicals (especially methylparabins, found in most skin and body products, including lotions, creams, shampoos, conditioners); spray nets, hair permanents, hair color, chemical hair removers; make-up; nail polish and remover; antiperspirants; bubble bath and shower gels; sunscreen; body powder; and toothpaste.

Art materials: Most paints (except for poster and watercolor); pastels, spray glue and spray paint, solvents and dyes.

Household objects: Furniture made of particle board with wood veneer finishes gas off formaldehyde; rugs and mattresses laced with chemical fire retardants or chemical sealers to protect against stains; living close to cell towers or electricity pole transformers; cell phones; electromagnetic radiation; and radon.

Air quality: Living in cities; near freeways; house mold; and toxic building materials like asbestos insulation, and particle board or plywood cabinets.

If using any products containing toxic chemicals, treat them cautiously by wearing gloves, having good ventilation or wearing a mask, and using an air purifier at home and in the workplace. Houseplants, such as spider plants or Boston fern, can be of help as they absorb chemicals, especially formaldehyde.

Better yet, less toxic products should be substituted when possible. Due to the huge demand of the health food business, many of these products can be purchased in a less toxic form or with no toxicity at all. Again, read labels! Be informed! And be aware that many products advertise as organic or natural and still contain problematic chemicals.

Because of the tremendous amount of toxic chemicals found in common everyday items, it is our own individual responsibility to check those products and read labels in order to maintain the least toxic environment and lifestyle possible in this sadly polluted world.

20

In Retrospect

*L*OOKING BACK OVER MY LIFE AND TRYING TO understand my illness, I don't think I will ever truly know the exact underlying cause. More than anything, my guess is that it probably was a combination of genetic potential (having two relatives with lymph cancers); a clogging diet contributing to a sluggish lymphatic system most of my life; deep-rooted fears; and karma (if such a thing exists — not as punishment, but as an opportunity to develop greater wisdom, compassion and healing resources). And the final straw, I believe, was being around carcinogenic chemicals for years in my art field, most especially exposure to fumes from the ink press six months before diagnosis, and cleaning up flea powder two years before. All of this, plus suppressing symptoms with medication every time I had a cold or minor illness and missing that opportunity for cleansing and repair in order to maintain a balanced, healthful state.

I truly have been given a second chance, and I treat myself with much greater care and awareness. What a gift to be able to do that! It has been a miraculous healing process, yet it is also very much a case of cause and effect—of creating supportive conditions that allow the depths of my body's healing ability to carry out the work for which it is intended, so that it may function at its highest potential, so that I may function at mine.

"Miracles do happen; they are not interruptions
or violations of the laws of nature or physics,
rather they are confirmations of laws
beyond physics and affirmations of the deeper depths
of nature's law."

Linda Goodman

Related Reading

For a wealth of inspiring stories about healing cancer, type in **Cancer Healing** *at Amazon.com.*

NON-TOXIC PRODUCT DIRECTORY
Home Safe Home by Debra Lynn Dadd,
Penguin Putnam Inc., 1997

WONDERFUL HEALING STORIES
Living Proof: A Medical Mutiny by Michael Gerin-Tosh,
Scribner, 2003
To Health: The New Humanistic Oncology
by Jacob Zighelboim, MD., Booksurge.com
A Cancer Therapy: Results of Fifty Cases by Max Gerson, MD,
Station Hill Press, Inc, 1958
*Embrace, Release, Heal: An Empowering Guide to
Talking About, Thinking About, and Treating Cancer*
by Leigh Fortson, Sounds True Publishing

NUTRITIONAL INFORMATION

Fasting and Eating for Health: A Medical Doctor's Program for Conquering Disease by Joel Fuhrman, MD, St. Martin's Griffin Press, 1995

Natural Strategies for Cancer Patients by Russell L. Blaylock, MD, Kensington Books, 2003

HEALING SUPPORT

Journey Through Cancer: Healing and Transforming the Whole Person by Jeremy R. Geffen, MD, Three Rivers Press, 2006

Skills for Awakening by Ram Giri, PHD, http://skillsforawakening.com

The Conscious Cancer Journey by Melanie Brown, www.consciouscancerjourney.com

DREAMS AND HEALING

Avalanche by W. Brugh Joy, MD, Ballantine Books, 1992

Healing Dreams: Exploring the Dreams That Can Transform Your Life by Marc Ian Barasch, The Berkley Publishing, 1992

VISUALIZATION

The Healing Journey by O. Carl Simonton, MD,
Brenda Hampton, and Reid Henson,
Author's Choice Press, 1992

Getting Well Again by O. Carl Simonton, MD,
James Creighton, PHD, Stephanie Matthews Simonton,
and Stephanie Matthews,
Mass Market Paperback, 1992

Healing from Cancer—Audio CD (Oct. 1, 2005)
by Emmett Miller, MD

Healing Visualizations:
Creating Health Through Imagery
by Dr. Gerald Epstein,
Bantam Books, 1989

Rituals of Healing: Using Imagery for Health and
Wellness by Barbara Dossey and Jeanne Achterberg,
Bantam Books, 1994

PRAYER

MAP—Medical Assistance Program
by Machaelle Small Wright,
Perelandra, 1994

About the Author

Dale Figtree, PhD has been a nutritional health practitioner for over twenty-seven years and an artist since childhood. She has a private nutritional consulting practice in Santa Barbara, California, and taught "The Basics of Nutrition" for several years at the Santa Barbara College of Oriental Medicine. Dr. Figtree presents nutritional seminars throughout the United States and Europe, and is the author of two books, **Eat Smarter: The Smarter Choice for Healthier Kids** and **Health after Cancer**, and the DVD/video, **The Joy of Nutrition**.